Alzheimer's and Dementia . . .

This Ugly Disease

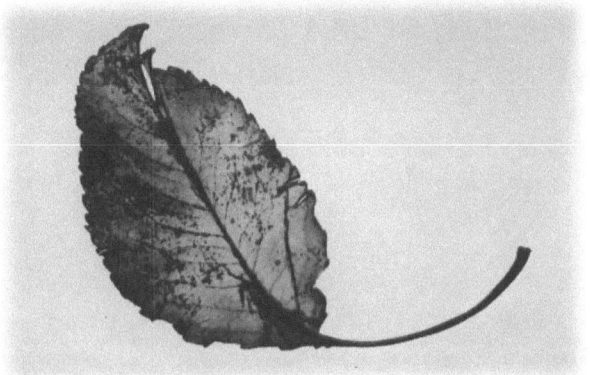

*A Caregiver's Journey into
Pain, Anguish and Hope*

By Donald Zoller
Foreword by Virginia Katz

"Alzheimer's and Dementia . . . This Ugly Disease:

A Caregiver's Journey into Pain, Anguish and Hope"

Copyright © 2016, 2019 by Donald Zoller

Bible quotations are taken from the Holy Bible, English Standard
Version. Copyright © 2011 by Crossway Bibles.

To Beverley

(1942–2016)

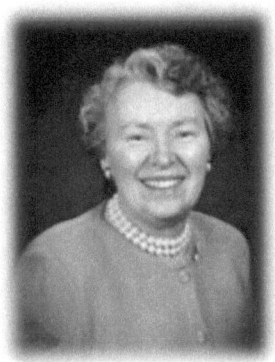

A rose in my garden I never knew
Until the day I smelled its fragrance,
Beheld its beauty—Placed it gently in my hand.
Now, precious; it is but a memory of something past
But never forgotten.
                                           —Donald Zoller

The story of my journey as a caregiver is dedicated to my wife, Beverley. For over 55 years she has been at my side as wife, friend and confidant. Although these last few years have been challenged by this ugly disease, she is no less a wonderful, adorable and lovable woman who is the joy of my life and a source of special blessing. The strength of her faith and her walk with God have provided inspiration and encouragement to many, including her three sons and, of course, her husband. Thank you, Beve.

A Word of Thanks

My journey as a caregiver has been overwhelming and exhausting, to say the least. But, along the way, several have helped and need a special "thank you." Their help makes an impossible task *possible*.

As Beverley entered the dark days of dementia, our home group from our church in Kansas City provided their love and help. We have been encouraged by their kindness, sentiment cards and especially by their prayers. *Charlotte Adelsperger*, a member of our group, spent many prayerful hours with Bev when I needed a break—a beautiful heart and a wonderful help. *Charlotte,* an accomplished writer, also provided much-needed professional guidance for the book. *Howard Russell* guided us to the right neurologist to accurately assess Bev's condition—thanks, Howard. In addition to these, several from the Sojourners Sunday School class prayed and expressed their love and support in so many practical ways.

After making the move to Texas, several helped Bev during her downward journey into dementia. Arc Home Health, Hospice Select and Envoy Hospice extended their valuable services—their help is deeply appreciated. The staff at House "B" of Mustang Creek Estates, Bev's new home, also needs a special word of thanks for their relentless and self-sacrificing efforts to make the memory-loss residents comfortable, safe and peaceful.

A special thanks to *Carol Stainer* who connected with us in Macy's—a wonderful godly lady who makes a prayerful effort each day to meet someone new—like us. As a couple of newbies in town, she introduced us to a local home group, which has been especially supportive. She also shared with us that her son had recently passed away with dementia.

Then there is *Joseph Lenard*, my friend and co-author of *The Last Shofar!* (2014) who helped immeasurably in editing the book. A special thanks goes to *Rod Laughlin*, a servant-pastor, teacher and author of the *Readable Bible*—and friend. Rod provided valuable insights into what words would best touch the heart of the reader.

Of course, I want to mention *Virginia Katz*, whose husband was at the same memory care facility as Bev. He came to memory care the day after Beverley and passed away the day after Bev did. *Virginia* graciously wrote the Foreword to this book. Thank you, *Virginia*.

Our three sons: *Greg*—and his family, who have given much by way of hands-on support, and *Graham* and *Garth*—although both living at a distance, have also given in loving tangible ways to their mother and me. I am fully blessed to have them as my sons.

Finally, my deepest thanks belong to the *Lord*, who kept me going, constantly reminding me of His faithfulness, love and forgiveness—I needed all the reminding I could get. Before and after Bev's move to the memory care, I had three eye surgeries—all on the same eye. Emergency surgery restored temporary blindness—the eye healed and so did the vision. He is the One who kept me from depression, and energized me to put together this booklet—all in the space of four *interrupted* weeks with only one working eye. It's really His book! *An amazing miracle—thank you, Lord!*

Just a Note

Alzheimer's is commonly understood as a unique and mentally debilitating fatal disease. Whereas, most people view "dementia" as only somewhat related to Alzheimer's. However, medically understood, Alzheimer's is, in fact, a subset of dementia. Correctly understood, dementia is the larger umbrella within which Alzheimer's resides as well as several other forms of dementia. But, for the purpose of this book we will keep the commonly accepted understanding intact—simply using "Alzheimer's" and "dementia" interchangeably.

Table of Contents

Foreword

By Virginia Katz
A Friend and Fellow Caregiver

There are many articles and books written on the subject of Alzheimer's and dementia, explaining the progression of the disease and "what may be expected to come." They also talk about being a caregiver, offering advice—*including warnings,* and about how important it is for the caregiver to take care of their own health in this process. But, as someone who has lived with a spouse suffering from this horrible disease for about five years, this is the *first and only book* I have read that made me feel I had not been alone in my journey of mixed emotions, frustrations, and feelings of guilt when I became angry and absolutely exhausted throughout this ordeal.

I had recently come to a point where I felt totally helpless and that there was no "light at the end of the tunnel." No matter how much I had tried to keep my loved one at home to the end of this disease, I had nothing left to give physically or mentally, and I had to find a place where he could be cared for and be safe. I still felt sadness and guilt, and questioned myself if I had done the right thing.

After reading Don Zoller's, *This Ugly Disease,* I am truly now at peace with myself and have come to the realization that I made the most loving decision I could have made *for* my spouse. I hope that others who are dealing with this ugly disease as a caregiver will read this book and realize they, too, are not alone. I am truly grateful that he shared his experience and so many feelings in order to help others like myself.

A Beginning Word

This booklet may not be for you. In fact, many would not fully understand it since they have not walked the painful path nor experienced the tortuous anguish of the journey. What I am putting into words, unlike a clinical "how to" manual on caregiving or even expressing concerns of an empathic observer, emerges out of the depths of my experience as a frustrated and exhausted caregiver. You who are on this journey with me, holding the hand of a loved one afflicted by the ravages of Alzheimer's or dementia, will know immediately the words I use to describe our common experience as caregivers.

My purpose is to talk about the shared experiences of the daily and often unrelenting struggles of a caregiver that rarely are discussed—at least in polite company. I also want to encourage you along this thorny and painful journey of trying so hard to meet the increasing needs and demands of those we love but who are quickly slipping away from us. The challenges are real. The journey is hard. *Very hard! But we are not alone!*

I have drawn freely from my own experiences and those of others. In my conversations with other caregivers and from my readings of several books and articles, I have discovered two unexpected things:

First, I am not alone on this path of giving care—giving care until it hurts, *and it does hurt a lot!* Many, yes untold millions, are dealing with the exact same challenges; sometimes successfully, but mostly not. Most of us are hidden from view, bearing the load alone—not even our closest family members and friends *fully* understand or appreciate the magnitude of the weight we carry every single hour of the day, even while the rest of the world sleeps.

Second, many excellent available resources fall short for those of us who are struggling with caregiving. Often, they fail to adequately touch the shedding of our tears of anguish, guilt, anger and desperation—the agony of experiencing daily our loved one who is being removed from us by *this ugly disease*. None adequately describe the heavy load carried by the caregiver who is desperately trying to meet the need of the person they love, even as they see them sinking deeper and deeper into a *memory lost*. Nor do these resources fully enter into the deeper issues of what we do or don't do for our loved one when life-decisions are forced upon us. The bottom line of our heart-wrenching struggles often come down to this: *"What is the loving thing to do?"*

In answering this question, we first see ourselves as the *Unqualified to Do the Impossible (Chapter 1)*. A look at *Simple Beginnings (Chapter 2)* is my personal story, but could be any caregiver's story—even your story. *Challenged Beyond our Ability (Chapter 3)* becomes our new reality. When we ask, *Who's Around to Help? (Chapter 4)* we have taken the first step toward answering the question. At some point, however, each of us must face the inevitable, *What is the loving thing to do? (Chapter 5)* Soon we discover that *Letting Go* and *Waiting (Chapters 6 &7)* can present new and unexpected challenges. *As a Final Word,* I have added a few thoughts about *Faith*—for me, a "must have" for my journey. As an addendum, A *Lost Ring – The End of A Journey* is included to share with you my last hours with Beverley. *Not an easy thing to write!*

As a fellow sojourner, join me as we travel into a crazy upside-down world of caregiving that is never simple or straightforward. What seems to be right often turns out to be wrong, and the paths we choose we often find go in circles. Adding to our misery, we no longer comprehend the words of our loved one—they make no sense either to our ears or mind. Our dark emotions rise up like formidable mountains of ugliness that get in the way of being the loving caregiver we know we should be. Welcome to our own special, *"Alice in Wonderland"—a story that is rarely told, understood or even listened to.*

This Ugly Disease

Chapter 1

Unqualified to Do the Impossible

I really don't like job interviews, but you have to do them if you want the job. When interviewing, employers usually pay special attention to experience, skills and suitability of the prospective employee, i.e., can they handle the demands of the job? Looking forward, will the applicant and the employer experience a measure of success as an outcome from this new job? I think it is safe to say, however, that none of us as caregivers remember applying or being interviewed for our job. Somehow, we seemed to have missed that process altogether.

If you are like me, many of you probably are of an age where the finish line of life is coming into view. You spent a lot of effort—and money, to get an education. You found a job, or perhaps more than one, during your employment years. Perhaps you were married and raised a family—you dealt with all the challenges, disappointments, and, yes, sometimes heartaches each of these phases of life presented.

Let's face it, with all of the scars and hard knocks many of us experienced throughout our maturing years, we were prepared to settle back and move comfortably into the last quarter of life. We looked forward to sharing our life stories with family and friends, settling into our favorite retirement location, playing golf, or some other activity, and traveling, at least this is what all the literature seems to suggest. But, seemingly out of nowhere, we are handed a new job, one for which we are not qualified to do—one that neither success nor remuneration can be found in the job description.

Nothing in our education, job experience, or raising a family prepared us to be caregivers. We had no innate skills or aptitudes that would assure our success. In fact, the truth be known, most of us are terribly unsuccessful most of the time as caregivers. Any measure of feeling successful in caring for a loved one with Alzheimer's or dementia soon evaporates with time. Eventually, from the depths of our being, we literally cry out—sometimes yell, *"I can't do this anymore!"* And yet, the demands for giving care to the one we love continue to force us forward to new levels of desperation where our cry, *"I can't do this anymore!"* gets loud enough that at times we may wonder if the neighbors can hear us. Will they call 911?

As the volume and intensity of our inability to adequately care for our loved one increase, we soon realize the utter impossibility of our task. Often, we collapse with complete exhaustion, exasperation and with a horrible feeling of defeat. The reality is that we feel this drama is ours and ours alone. No one is around to witness what we are experiencing. We might imagine that our dramatic episodes would make a great reality TV series, but, alas, there's no one around to see it. In those times, we are alone, sharing our tears and anguish with no one else.

Without training or preparation for caregiving, most of us would say that we are handed one of the toughest jobs on earth. Not many of us are equipped to be a Mother Teresa or a Florence Nightingale in giving care to the needy. In speaking with several people who see themselves as having strong emotional and physical caring attributes they shared with me that they, too, eventually hit the wall and crashed with the reality that this constant and ever-increasing 24/7 caregiving is beyond human endurance.

A neighbor whose wife has dementia shared with me that during his working years he headed up large corporations with all of its challenges of managing production and people. During business downturns he had the difficult job of letting hundreds of people go— *"That was really a tough thing to do."* However, he said that providing care for his wife for the past three years has been the toughest job he has ever had. It isn't easy! We will talk about this a little more in Chapter Three, *Challenged Beyond our Ability.*

I think we can all agree that in our new role as caregivers we are *unqualified to do the impossible.* Yes, many of us receive praises from family and friends for the wonderful self-sacrificing job we are doing in caring for our loved one. They may even say, *"We just don't know how you do it!"* (Nor do we!). And yet, we find it difficult to enlist the help of some who may find it easier to toss accolades than taking the helm for a couple of days while we recover our sanity. Welcome to my world!

So, what have we learned about the job of caregiving? We know it is an exhausting and overwhelming job that few, if any, really want at the *end of the day*. It comes with an abundance of uncompensated labor filled with thankless 24/7 hours of hardship and heartbreak. Caregiving takes a terrible toll on our own personal health with high levels of stress that affect body, mind and spirit. It quickly drains our buckets of physical, mental, emotional and spiritual resources. We soon find we have little to give except orders—I call this phase the "barking dog" syndrome.

The greatest unknown about the job is the degree of appreciation our loved one has toward the care he or she is receiving from us. From all appearance there is none—something we dare not think about too long. *Caregiving is the toughest and loneliest job in the world!*

Why then do we continue doing it? Why do we continue in a role for which we are unqualified and for which positive outcomes are impossible? If it is your spouse, perhaps it is remembering a wedding vow—a promise, *"for better, for worse, for richer, for poorer, in sickness and in health, until death do us part."* Maybe it is less formal, simply a commitment of the heart to show love to the one whose life you shared for so many years—wonderful memories of a beautiful life together. It may be hard for some observers to understand our level of commitment. The Apostle Paul in writing to the church at Corinth talked about it this way,

Love bears all things, believes all things,
hopes all things, endures all things.
I Corinthians 13:7

Chapter 2

Simple Beginnings

This Chapter is about my personal journey as a husband and caregiver to my wife, Beverley, who was afflicted with vascular dementia sometimes referred to as *Vascular Cognitive Impairment*. In this story you may find many parallels to your own experience. The details may be unique, but the final outcome is the same.

The Wife I Knew

Beverley was full of energy, active and forthright—without hesitation she told you what she was thinking regardless of the social setting. Having a wide range of interests, she taught women's Bible studies, mentored several women one-on-one ›and was deeply committed to international mission work. Faith was her strength and God, her companion and friend.

Bev's cooking was *to die for*, constantly preparing wonderful meals and baking fantastic cookies—her favorites were sugar and chocolate chip cookies. With a fluent knowledge of plants, including the Latin names for each and every flora and fauna in her garden, her exotic *cottage gardens* covered every piece of bare earth in sight.

Oh yes, Bev raised a family of three loving sons; seeing each of them through college with at least one master's degree. For over 25 years, she lovingly cared for her mother, Jean. As a devoted homemaker all her married life, Bev was my life-partner and intimate confidant for the first 51 of our 55 years together. Truly a remarkable woman! She is *still* my lovable and adorable wife!

Early Signs

It began simply enough. Early on in our marriage we were aware that dementia was pervasive in the family gene pool on Bev's father's side, but we really didn't name it or see it as an early warning sign. In time, it became obvious that something was not quite right with her father—forgetting things and "fogging" in and out of reality. All her uncles, aunts and cousins behaved in similar ways. Bev's brother also now shows signs of this ugly disease (He has since passed away, 2018). I guess we concluded, *"That was them, not us."* Sometimes, when you are busy with life you don't always integrate the obvious. Maybe, it was just our expression of denial.

When Bev moved into her forties, certain behaviors were obvious to our sons—when you live too close to the forest you don't always see the trees, which was my case with spotting early signs. Whenever she was still and listening, she began twitching her mouth—a little strange, but I assumed it was just a small affectation. Since it was not a big thing, I let it pass without comment. No big deal . . . I thought! Occasionally, she would begin to forget people's names and places—all very recoverable with promptings from me, and life seemingly moved on normally.

Simple Beginnings No More

In her early sixties Bev had a series of fender-benders with her car—nothing serious, except she could not remember how they happened. One event, however, brought the obvious to a head. Although thankfully no one was injured, she totaled her car. Eventually, with signs of diminishing attention to driving, we sold her car. Having only one car with me as the sole driver was okay with her—she never did like to drive anyway. However, looking back, I now can see that this decision to have just one car was the beginning of my becoming an *active* caregiver. She still needed to get to events and go shopping, but now she was dependent on me to meet those needs.

I was still free to go off on my own to meet with the guys for coffee, get a haircut and take care of other personal needs. She was safe enough to leave alone at home and answer the phone if I called. But her ability to communicate clearly on the phone began to diminish. Her response to a call was to immediately give the "local weather report" or some other unrelated information. Soon, even this was reduced to only a few, often-unintelligible words. With one exception—her use of the credit card.

Bev used her credit card generously and with great clarity when placing phone orders for flowers and clothes from catalogues. Up to this point she managed the household budget, but for obvious reasons I could see that this was not going to work. I decided the time had come to move the budget from a paper process to the computer. This allowed me to see and to manage the income and expenses. It took several months to bring order out of unsupervised spending. Bev still recorded expenses in the checkbook registry, but in time even this task became erratic and difficult for her to do.

The Death of Mother Jean

Jean had a sharp "don't mess with me" mind, even at 102. It was her body that was wearing out. Jean lived with us during her final years and eventually passed away at 102, two months shy of her 103rd birthday! A few months before she passed away, Jean called me into her room and said, "We've got to talk! I am very concerned about Beverley. I think she needs to see a neurologist." That got my attention. After some unsatisfying starts, we finally found a neurologist that understood Bev's condition and made the appropriate tests—MRI, blood work and other tests. The result came back. Bev had *moderate vascular dementia*. But, I am getting ahead of my story.

During the time of trying to find the right medical help for Bev, her mother passed away. Bev did not show any expression of grief, sorrow or loss at her mother's bedside at the time of death at the hospice home or at her funeral—or any time since. The absence of grief and loss was especially strange considering how very close they were to each other. They were the best of friends always laughing and talking with each other. But, it was as though Bev was the attending nurse or simply a detached attendee at a funeral of someone she did not know. When asked about her deceased mother, she had only a short mantra, *"She liked to bake pies and she worked in a boys' summer camp."*

The Downward Journey

Forgetting how to operate the microwave and leaving on the top burners of the stove, forgetting how to put together ingredients to bake her favorite cookies, which ended in uneatable disasters, or leaving out pieces and parts of her special and family-loved recipes—all led me to see my next role as caregiver—managing the kitchen, including, eventually, "cooking" the meals. As a man, who stayed out of the kitchen, often by orders from the cook, what did I possibly know about this strange part of the house? About this time, Bev also lost her passion for gardening. The gardening catalogues still arrived in the mail but were put aside and piled high in a corner of the kitchen.

Hallucinating and seeing "talking" faces in the ceiling fan became common, mitigated somewhat by the Exelon Patch and Namenda prescribed by her neurologist. Unfinished sentences also became common, often repeating my words spoken to her rather than responding to them. I had to learn to decouple complex questions, making them separate questions and very "pithy." Soon her words became few—some I did not even understand. Dialogue, for the most part, became a thing of the past.

We moved from Kansas to Texas in late 2014 to be closer to the grandchildren and to reduce the size and footprint of our home—to 1500 square feet with only four rooms. But disorientation was almost daily—not knowing where to find the bedroom or bathroom. All of this was compounded with her frequent wanderings—always wanting to respond to the person outside the house who was calling her name—in her head. These wanderings were particularly "popular" after going to bed—*sundowner's syndromes.* Special locks were installed on the exterior doors to keep her from wandering outside the house while I was attempting to get some sleep.

She moved with determination and strength, almost super-human strength. Nothing seemed to stop her. She was in a different reality, one that cannot be reasoned with or easily redirected. This only added to my exasperation. One thing that had a calming influence was watching "I Love Lucy" reruns at two in the morning.

Eventually, Bev lost the ability to get from "A" to "B." She knew what each looked like but her ability to get from "here to there" was gone. Routinely, I dressed her and many times manned the "mop and pail brigade," common with incontinency. She eventually lost awareness of days and time—getting ready for church at all hours of the night. I regularly retrieved her from the shower and other bathroom needs as she lost her sense of time and understanding why she was even in the bathroom.

Where We Are Now

During the past two years, I have been promoted to a full-time caregiver with all the challenges and anguish that go with the job—we'll look at that in the next chapter. Beverley, with her posture stooped and speaking little, now resides comfortably in a memory care facility. She seems to be nearing the end of a statistically seven-year journey for most people with vascular dementia. But only God knows when it will be time for her to go home—*truly home.*

Remember, a sickness or disease, no matter how ugly and hard it is to manage, can never sever a relationship forged in love.

Now It's Your Turn

I have given you a template. Write out your story—your journey with your loved one. This will be your "Chapter 2." You can use similar subtitles to help you organize your thoughts. It may be a little painful; you may need some help from a family member or close friend, but write! It will be wonderful therapy. You will find it a meaningful release.

Chapter 3

Challenged Beyond our Ability

I never tire of watching the guy or gal scaling an extreme vertical rock face, even with overhangs, all without any external support, safety ropes, or even pinions. Their ability to hug a vertical rock surface is amazing. Constantly challenged, their faultless ability and fearless tenacity are climaxed with a victory-wave at the top, making it an exciting and nail- biting TV event. But, I often wonder about the ones who don't make it. You know, the ones whose hold on a rock fails or whose footing gives way—the ones that aren't talked about or shown on adventure TV. Then I think of the many, so many, who are not making it in caring for their loved ones with Alzheimer's or dementia. Like those who don't give the victory-wave, we will never be talked about or seen on *adventure TV.*

Usually, we are far up on *the rock face* when it happens. Fighting to hang on, griping onto everything we can, yet we lose it— big time! It's tough, this business of caregiving. We may try to present a stoic and easy-going face to family and friends, but they can see the stress lines, they can hear the fatigue in our voice. When asked, *"How is it going?"* often our response is the biggest lie we tell: *"Just fine,"* hoping the conversation ends with that. Or, maybe it is out of kindness that we deflect the truth, thinking that they don't have the time to listen or really don't want to know about the *horrors of war* we face every day.

The extremes of *this ugly disease* are legend. From quite docile behaviors to highly aggressive ones and everything in between—all are characterized in some measure by what most of us see as erratic, irrational behaviors. Words that connect to nowhere, forgetfulness, disorientation, wanderings—particularly at night when behavior gets truly *wild—sundowner's syndromes.* Breaking things, putting things in the cupboard that eventually spoil because they should have been in the frig, regularly watering faux flowers resulting in water-soaked furniture, etc. Yes, invite family and friends to come around then and they will hear and see the real battle. According to the Alzheimer's Association, many caregivers don't make it—they die before those they are caring for.

Deep sleep and long showers are not in the job description of a caregiver. One eye and one ear open 24/7 is never-ending. It's more than just being on-call. It's rigorous duty all the time. Most night watchmen get paid for what they do, but not us. Noises in the night, or sounds that should not be heard during the day are alerts to us that something is amiss and needs our immediate attention, if not intervention. Without pay or gratuity, without a thank you from the one we love, and nothing but exhaustion, we do what is needed.

Then there are those feelings—feelings that produce high levels of sustained stress over a long period of time. Where do they come from? They are not part of us, normally. Or, are they? They are ugly and upon reflection we want no part of them. But there they are: anger, hate, cursing and frustration—all produce a lot of crying and yelling. Our anguish is compounded by our guilt for behaving and speaking the way we do. And the truth is that our loved ones cannot help themselves, and may not even know why we are making so much noise. How many times have we struggled with feeling terribly remorseful and guilty? How many times have we sought forgiveness for our behavior?

You, with your terrible thoughts and feelings that deluge your mind and burst forth in less than kind words—*you* are normal as a caregiver for a loved one with Alzheimer's or dementia. You are experiencing what I, and millions of others are experiencing. Forgive yourself for being less than you thought you were. You did not realize that you were not qualified, that you were unprepared, and that there are challenges none of us are up to.

There isn't a caregiver yet—and these are some of the nicest people you would ever want to meet—who hasn't had all these feelings in the dark times of their experience. You are not alone with your feelings. You are just facing an inescapable *challenge beyond your ability*.

Let's take a moment to look at ourselves in the mirror—when we step out of the shower. What do we see? For most of us it is not a physique that would adorn the covers on popular magazines found at our local checkout counters. The truth is that our body is aging, not like cheese or good wine, but like dried fruit. The strengths and energies of body and mind are not what they used to be, even on a good day. Yet, we are called upon as caregivers to be herculean. We are to be a specimen of humanity that can easily handle a *"10-ton marshmallow"* that are loved ones can feel like when we need to navigate them safely to the toilet, into the shower, or moving them through the house.

This leads to a related and obvious subject—one that is high on every caregivers list, or should be—*falling*. How many times at night do we watch the bed posts, the dresser and bathroom fixtures as we try to navigate our *"10-ton marshmallow"* to keep him or her from falling. Maybe it isn't even night—daylight hours can be just as challenging. There is the "thump" that only a falling body can make. On such occasions we are usually in the next room—that's just the way it works out. Hearing the "thump," we hope and pray that they have not hit anything on their journey to the floor.

There they are, in a place and position where it is hard to imagine anyone would be—wedged between furniture and, as was the case with Bev, wedged between the garbage cans in the garage. You now are faced with the task of trying to get your loved one back on their feet. Did I mention that they are usually oblivious to their fall and cannot help you, *even a little bit*. Where there is a significant weight difference, with the one fallen weighing more than you, this is an even more daunting situation. It becomes a *challenge beyond our ability*. As many of us can attest, falling is always a very present danger for the loved one and the caregiver. Both can experience injuries that no one wants or needs.

We all struggle with caregiving, but as a man I think it is harder to be a caregiver—at least this is my take on it. Typically, the caregiving DNA is not normally found in men of my generation. A captain of industry, a leader, a manager of process and production, a warrior, and explorer, *but not a caregiver!* It must be acquired the hard way; learning patience beyond measure, self-sacrificing beyond reason and learning to be a forbearing "mother" of an adult two-year old. As I said, caregiving isn't easy for anyone, but as a man I found it well beyond my natural ability. But we do it anyway. Maybe there is something in our character development as men that we missed in the maturing years that is now forced upon us.

Sometimes, whether a man or woman, our temperament may make a difference in our approach to our loved ones. Those of us who are easy-going and laid-back may find it a *bit* easier to deal with irrational and erratic behaviors. Although I am sure that there are easy-going caregivers, I have yet to find one. But, for those of us who are at the other end of the temperament scale, say a "Type A" personality or, like myself, a perfectionist consumed by details that require everything to be right and in its right place, we suffer a lot more, and more quickly. However, eventually we all come to that place where we lose our grip on a loose rock on the cliff-face, and begin our fall into deep despair, crying out, "*I can't do this any more!*" That's when we are *challenged beyond our ability.*

When we admit that we are challenged beyond our ability, and there are no other options; when we are exhausted beyond our endurance, we begin the next phase of caregiving—we begin to look around for help.

Chapter 4

Who's Around to Help?

I like to dream. To gaze into the future of what might be. But not all dreams come true. This one did not. As I see it now, I had a naïve dream that I could provide care for Bev until *death do us part*, within the four walls of our home. Like most I said, *"I don't need help. I can do it."* But, when Bev's needs exceeded my dream, I decided that with *a little* outside help, I would still be able to keep her at home to the end.

As this chapter reveals, I couldn't even do that. I soon found that even with friends and family, with all their love and good intentions, even with additional professional care, I could not do what eventually needed to be done.

Someone has said that we do not need help until *we really need help!* Being the stoics we often try to be, looking around for help—serious help doesn't cross our minds until we have finally, once for all, declared for the last time, *"I can't do this anymore! I need help!"* Even Mother Teresa had help—she had a whole clinic of helpers.

Have you ever thought that maybe caregiving was *never supposed* to be a "me-only" job? Maybe, caregiving, when it comes to Alzheimer's or dementia, means more than one. I don't know if the books on the subject of caregiving really talk about it in this way. But the fact is we often try to make it a one-person job, ours. That just does not work.

People, in their concern for our health as caregivers, drop hints about seeking help—from somewhere. *"That's okay. I can manage it,"* is our typical response. No, you can't! Many times, we reject the obvious and deny what is seen clearly by others. This was me for a long time *(too long)*—until it was forced on me, little by little.

First to arrive was a home-health company, encouraged by our doctor. Then it started—all these people (actually only three) *invading* my home. A registered nurse and two therapists: a physical therapist and a speech therapist who consumed the better part of a perfectly well-orchestrated week for several hours each week. When they came, I retreated into the next room while they worked with Beverley.

Let me pause here to insert some information that might help in understanding *Medicare* when it comes to home health, skilled nursing facilities, and doctors, generally. These are medical professionals whose job it is to make people "well" or at least provide a medically stable condition. With ailments that are not going to get better, but continue to get worse—such as Alzheimer's and dementia—home health, skilled nursing facilities, and doctors do not work. At best, these efforts are part of the Medicare program designed to get the patient better, hopefully in a matter of months. Therefore, extended home health wasn't going to be productive for Bev, or for anyone with this ugly disease.

Home health continued for about two months. As directed by Medicare regulations, they discontinued service. Soon thereafter another company called. This time it was in-home *hospice care*. At the time, I thought had to clarify that Beverley had no prospects of dying soon and that perhaps hospice care was a bit premature. No, they assured me. In-home hospice care is for anyone who is diagnosed as having a progressive and incurable disease, such as Alzheimer's or dementia.

As the name implies, in-home hospice has a single option for care. It is called *palliative care*, meaning care with no resuscitation, feeding tubes, or anything else that could represent "heroics." In-home hospice care can continue for years—as long as the patient shows evidence of decline determined every 60 days by a visiting hospice doctor (MD). Hospice care is regulated by a Do Not Resuscitate (DNR) order signed by the doctor. Medicare covers in-home hospice care, but under a different program than home health—yes, a whole new set of forms to complete! Just what you need!

If in-home hospice care is the preferred choice, Medicare requires all medical issues be handled through the hospice nurse and subsequently through the hospice doctor (MD). To say it another way, when you have in-home hospice, the doctors you are currently using for medical needs must be terminated. Dentist and eye doctors are okay, but even these eventually will cease once your loved one is no longer ambulatory. Once you make the decision to place your loved one into in-home hospice care, Medicare will help you, but it doesn't want to pay for redundant or *philosophically* conflicting services.

Remember, these are two different worlds. Doctors *outside* the in-home hospice care system seek to make the patient well or, at best, stable. They will use every means that is reasonable and available to them medically to make that happen.

In-home hospice, funded by Medicare, seeks *the comfort, safety and peace* of the patient—not to get better, but to live the remaining days of their life in a medically *passive* state, letting the body do what it will do over time until death. By the way, don't be surprised if the hospice doctor suggests that you get rid of the Exelon Patch and Namenda prescriptions. In time they lose their effectiveness, and besides you'll be saving lots of money on those two drugs alone. Hospice will provide medications, but only those that reasonably promote the comfort, safety and peace of the patient.

Having passed an initial assessment, Beverley became enrolled under in-home hospice care. It has a team of five: a registered nurse who visits once a week—but is also on-call 24/7, a nurse's assistant who comes every morning Monday through Friday to get Bev washed— including showers, dressed, and groomed; makes the bed and generally gets her ready for breakfast. The team also supports a social worker and chaplain who make regular visits, and a hospice doctor (MD) who makes in-home visits every two months. Medicare, under in-home hospice, pays for most everything needed to aid in palliative care, including medications, protective clothing, equipment, etc. There will be differences in how care is administered in your home and how it is handled in a memory care facility. There are also differences between hospice companies, but generally you will find they are basically trying to achieve the same thing. Pick the one that best meets your needs.

Although meeting some of my personal needs as a caregiver, in-home hospice was limited in caring for Beverley. The only relief I had was about an hour each morning from Monday through Friday when the aide arrived at the front door. My physical and emotional batteries were still running dangerously dry! I then decided to hire a *home companion care* service that specialized in caring for dementia patients. This gave me two four-hour segments each week that allowed me to do whatever needed to be done, even if it was to go down to the community center to work out or have a cup of coffee, while Bev was being cared for.

However, even with all this help it did not cover the growing demands Bev's dementia was placing on my ability to care and manage her. The nightly *sundowner's* events were increasing and I was getting less and less sleep. I keenly felt for her safety and my inability to adequately care for her physically and emotionally. This was real—I now needed *major* help!

To shorten the story, what finally answered Bev's need and mine as a caregiver was found only two and half miles from home. It was a memory care facility that was non-institutional (individual cottages) and comparatively budget friendly for the pocketbook. It provided palliative care (remember, memory care is all about palliative care) in a home-like environment for about 15 residents within each of four buildings. It was also a place where I could redirect my current in-home hospice staff to continue working with Bev. As great as it is, is it the perfect place? No, but I am learning that the word, "perfect," doesn't really exists for those caring for those afflicted with Alzheimer's and dementia. See more about this in Chapter Six, *Letting Go.*

To sum up, all these "helps" took place within a five-month period—how quickly this ugly disease travels! Yes, I needed help, but for the most part all this help came looking for me. It came knocking on my door. It may be different for you, but looking back, I will say the indicators are all around you, telling you that *you need help*. My guess, you probably need help *now*.

I am fully aware that getting help, if getting help is even in your plan, is an extremely personal matter. Timing, family, budget, and location—all and more, are factors to consider. Most of us don't have *Long-Term Care Insurance* to help cover costs, and *asking other family members*, particularly children, to help financially can be awkward, but sometimes absolutely necessary to do what is best for providing help for "Mom" or "Dad." Every family situation is different.

Initially, I would go directly either to an in-home hospice, and ask for an interview or assessment in your home; or get in touch with a memory care facility to gather the information you need to help form your decision. Your approach may vary depending on your location.

A good rule of thumb that somebody wiser than me said, "What was the condition of your loved one six months ago? What is it today? What will it look like six months from now? Will you be able to handle it then?" Wisely, make you decision today based on your expected need in six months. Most caregivers I have spoken to wondered why they waited six months before taking action. But there are other issues involved when considering what's the loving thing to do for our loved one. We'll look at some of these in the next chapter.

A list of resources I used, some mentioned in this book—some not—are noted at the back of the book.

Chapter 5

What's the Loving Thing to Do?

As caregivers, with all the challenges, issues and feelings—usually not pleasant ones, we deeply love the one who is in our care. I have a photo of Bev, the way she used to be, on my desk next to my computer. There are a lot of good memories coming from that photograph—51 years of them. In those memories, I have captured the person I love, and I still do love her after 55 years. It is just this blending of lives over a long period of time that brings each caregiver *eventually* to ask the question, *"What's the loving thing to do?"*

I really think that most caregivers have answered this question *in measured ways* from the first time they became aware that they had to give care to the one they loved, the one that had been a part of their life for so many years, and now, will no longer be the same. *"What is the loving thing to do?"* is seen over time in how we arranged the furniture, prepared the food, planned the daily schedule, etc. Yes, even removing the car keys, the credit cards and other items that could be harmful to them, and to you.

With the sincerest of intentions, the loving thing to do, we believed, was to keep them comfortable, safe and at peace in their own home, in the surroundings with which they were most familiar. But the heartache of every caregiver comes when this ugly disease does not cooperate with our best and most sincere intentions. When, at its extremes, the comfortable, safe and peaceful place we call home becomes a hell on earth. It becomes a nightmare scenario with our cries for help and our inability to continue life as it is. At his point, *"What is the loving thing to do?"* becomes a deeper and more profound question.

The question most likely will be answered in terms of relocating our loved one—a hard and almost unthinkable thought. Timing, family considerations, costs, location, type of care facility, etc., come flooding into my mind. But there is more. There is the stark reality that *your loved one will not be coming home again*. No more will they be sleeping next to you in bed or occupying the chair in the living room, watching TV with you, or sharing food at the table. No longer able to hold their hand in time of need. In some way, it is like death, *but not being dead*. This is what I mean when I say, *"What is the loving thing to do?"* takes on a deeper and more profound nature. It becomes the caregiver's ultimate question.

You as a caregiver may decide to stick it out to the end at home, come hell or high water. Even with some outside help, you decide you are going be the gallant warrior and continue on in the space where you are, whatever the residual cost and pain of doing so may be. I, and many others, with the deepest respect, salute you in your decision. Although your decision is a deeply personal one, seek out the counsel of others who can give you an objective opinion about your situation.

If, however, you decide the loving thing to do is to relocate them to a safer and more fitting place, then you have to consider the following options: If there are no immediate acute medical considerations, you may select a memory care facility or a skilled nursing facility. Just remember, as long as your loved one is in a memory care facility, no *direct* medical care is provided. If serious medical attention becomes necessary, memory care facilities, working with family and hospice care, if appropriate, will relocate the resident to the proper medical facility. That was the case with Beverley when three successive falls required hospital attention, and more forms to sign.

If palliative care is important to you, then going with an in-home hospice is the normal route. However, a hospice doctor must certify that your loved one is qualified to receive such care. But remember, whether a memory care or a skilled nursing facility is selected, the caregiver will pay *out-of-pocket* for non-medical care, a portion of which is reclaimable on you income tax as a long-term medical expense.

Let's get back to our question, *"What's the loving thing to do?"* Although not set in stone, the answer is nevertheless rather permanent.

One thing for sure, the loved one will not, in most cases, be returning home. Whatever is decided will affect not only your loved one *but you as well—for a long time.* Be careful not to substitute your personal feelings and preferences in place of doing what is best for your loved one, in the long term.

You need to ask, "What makes the most sense?" If you decide to relocate your loved one to memory care, will he or she receive better 24/7 care there than they would if they remained at home under your care? The answer may seem obvious, but it becomes, in my experience, more reaffirming after such a decision is made.

This may not be a complete answer to the question, *"What's the loving thing to do?"* but I hope it provides enough food for thought to clarify your thinking and to motivate you toward a positive course of action for your loved one. After you have made your decision, if it is to relocate your loved one outside of your home, realize that there is help available to make the transition easier. Contact your in-home hospice care, a memory care facility, or a skilled nursing facility. Also, the internet is a wonderful place to begin a search or investigate specific facilities.

The question, *"What is best for your loved one?"* really includes a second, but no less important question, *"What is best for you?"* That is, for your mental, emotional, physical and spiritual health. One of the most repeated questions I get from doctors, nurses and other professionals in the memory care community is, "How are you doing?"

It is not a casual question, but rather one that they sincerely want to know, in view of the stress load of caregiving, how am I holding up? There is with this question a probability that I am not doing all that great, which, in fact, is true. A high stress load for over two years took its toll on my health. When I came to the place where I needed to answer the question, "What is best for your loved one?" I also needed to answer the question, "What is best for you?" You see, we cannot take care of our loved one appropriately unless we are also taking care of ourselves. This eventually means getting professional caregiving help. As mentioned previously, caregivers who do not care for themselves often do not survive the one they are caring for.

Understand that you are truly loving your loved one by providing them with the best care possible, even if that care is given by someone other than you. When you reach the point that you are unable to provide what is needed, you continue to love them by letting others help. By letting others help, you are doing what is best for you as well as your loved one.

Chapter 6

Letting Go

A tornado warning sounds. Wind increases until, like the roar of a freight train, it plunges the house into blackness—and turmoil. A family emerges from a place of safety and looks on with a sense of bewilderment and loss—a tragedy to be sure. All they possessed is no more—it's gone! In a moment of time! Except for a few family photos they are able to recover from the debris, they no longer possess anything—it will all end up in the landfill. Or, maybe it's a Katrina-size hurricane with a total loss from flooding of everything we once had the day before. Fire can also render all you own into a pile of ashes—there is nothing left. Those who are resilient to tragedy, usually say, "it's all just stuff! Let it go! At least we are alive."

The truth is that most of us don't know much about this level of loss or *letting go* unless we have known the tragedy of a tornado, or some other totally devastating event. But, whatever the loss, most of us still find it very difficult letting go. If we have sent kids off to college we have had a little taste of what means to let go; or letting them go to forge a life of their own many miles from home. I am sure my parents felt that sense of loss and letting go when, shortly after graduating from high school, I got on that bus that took me away to a distant place—now under the care of the US Army.

In such moments we understood something about letting go and what it feels like to have places in our home no longer occupied—empty rooms, empty spaces that our loved one used to fill. But really, we like to hang on to things—and to the people that we love.

For caregivers, there comes a point in time when *letting go*—letting go of what we want to hold on to—is real and difficult. We want to keep our loved one safe and comfortable in their home—we don't want to let go of them!

But having made the decision to let someone else care for our loved one, it's now time to let them go. Letting go is hard, even though in the long run we know it's best for them. I want to suggest three levels of *letting go* that every caregiver must think about when they come to the decision to relocate their loved one.

First, when we move our loved one to a memory care facility, what we are really talking about is moving them out of their home and placing them into another environment, perhaps at some distance away. Such a decision is not only challenging logistically, but very emotional. They are moved by the family car or other special transportation with personal affects, minimal furniture and clothing. All of that is hard enough, but soon the busyness of getting them "moved in" is followed by a deep sense of *aloneness.* For the first time the word, *"alone"* takes on new meaning. They are over "there," and we are "here." For us, it is a defining moment of separation. Leaving our loved one behind, we get into the car, head for the driveway, and return to our home—*alone*!

We may struggle coming to peace with the idea of being alone, particularly if the previous years have been spent together in a happy and fulfilling relationship. As a caregiver, we are free at last, but the shadows of being alone are real. I know from my own experience, that there are moments of awareness—flashbacks of Bev's presence that seem very real to me—whether it is watching TV, at the table or in bed. For a moment, I sense she is there, but of course she isn't. We physically have let them go, but now we must deal with the lingering sense of *aloneness.* Our lingering emotion still wants to hang on to our loved one—not wanting to let go. I have experienced that eventually this inner conflict comes to peace with the realty of being alone, both physically and emotionally. Not perfectly, but tolerably. It's not easy. It is part of the *final* grieving process.

The next level of *letting go* has to do with control. When your loved one was with you at home, you controlled the environment. You did for them what you felt was best within the boundaries of your home. You took great pains to ensure that your loved one was safe, comfortable and at peace—it was pretty much under your control. But now, the job of controlling belongs to someone else. The care facility, where your loved one now lives, is in charge of controlling the "house," and the residents.

The care facility controls the environment, even little things like setting the thermostat, to make sure your loved one is safe, comfortable and at peace. But are they doing what you would do—in the *way* that you would do it? Probably not. But we need to let go of the thought that somehow, we can control that space. Although attention is given to your loved one, the focus is now upon *community*—others that share the same facility, the same space. What benefits all the residents controls the setting.

Perhaps you have observed, as I have, that the residents often wander in confusion and forget what room belongs to them. They may try to sleep in beds that do not belong to them; they may rummage through other people's personal affects, not knowing really what they are doing. At first, I was quite disturbed when I saw such behaviors. But I had to learn that this was part of living in community with other Alzheimer's and dementia residents. This was part of *letting go* of my control over the environment in which my loved one now lives.

Even while being cared for 24/7 by professional staff, your caregiver instinct will drive you to want to be at the side of your loved one every day, if possible. You want to remain in control. Although you may be able to do that in the beginning when they are first relocated to a care facility, in time your *daily* presence is not all that necessary. In fact, you could be getting in the way of achieving what you truly want for your loved one—a place where they are free of distraction, interruption and agitation. In sense, they are under new management.

Only you can assess how the frequency of your visits is affecting your loved one and the staff that is caring for them. As difficult as it may be, in time your visits and those of your family will increasingly mean more for you than for your loved one, especially if your loved one has come to a point of not recognizing you. It is a reality that is hard for some to accept. It is another level of *"letting go."*

The third level of *letting go* is more subtle, yet can be more impacting than the other two. Up to this point you had to let go of your loved one being in *a different place*, and in that place you had to let go of your *control*. Although you know that taking care of your loved one at home is not sustainable, you are faced with the fact that placing them into a care facility means you have put them into an environment that is *collectively* dealing with this ugly disease.

Even though we would like it to be otherwise, we know those affected by Alzheimer's or dementia do not get better. The movement of this disease is continually downward, moving at different rates for different people, but nonetheless downward. As a resident of a care facility, your loved one is now one among a group who *collectively* suffer from this ugly disease. These are the facts.

They are receiving a level of care that would be impossible for you to achieve at home. However, living among those whose journey is progressively downward, the hard question is, "Does this disease now progress at a faster rate than if my loved one were living at home?" Perhaps—maybe even probably! To make their lives manageable in a group setting, some things are removed from them and a new environment is substituted—a new, more confined living environment, interacting with the other residents, etc. All can be unsettling and cause a further decline in cognitive health. But, they will eventually adjust to the *rhythm* of the other members of the community. However, *our* adjustment to this new reality typically is longer and more difficult to accept.

So, where are we? *Letting go* means more than moving our loved one to *a different place*. With that, it also means that we must move away from being a direct caregiver to become, once again, a life-partner to our loved one. Then, we must let go of trying to *control their environment*—that's someone else's job now. And the tough one—letting go of their *lives*. What was ultimately unsustainable at home is being properly *(no, not perfectly)* handled in community—24/7. Things are different now!

". . . when you were young, you used to dress yourself and walk wherever you wanted, but when you are old, you will stretch out your hands, and another will dress you and carry you where you do not want to go." (John 21:18)

Chapter 7

Waiting

It seems that most of life, even from conception, is about *waiting*. From our earliest memories we were told we needed to wait for our birthday or Christmas or some other significant day. When we were in school, we learned to wait for our grades to be posted. We had to wait for that promotion at work. We wait for our car to be repaired. Now, a little older, we often wait to see our doctor and wait again for test results. For the discerning spouse or child of an Alzheimer's or dementia loved one, no place seems more about *waiting* than a memory care facility.

Once we place our loved one into memory care, we learn about waiting, and waiting and waiting. We often see it in the empty expressions on the faces of the residents—our loved one included. We see them aimlessly walking the circular corridors, each day, and every day, doing the same thing—waiting. Maybe it's just sitting for long hours staring into space, or confined to a bed. Sometimes *waiting* means waiting for the next meal, and the meal after that. Do our loved ones experience the passing of time, hence, *waiting?* The hard truth is that it is we who probably suffer the deep agony of waiting—*waiting for the inevitable to occur—waiting for the end of life* of our loved one.

During my initial meeting with the director of the memory care facility where Bev is now a resident, I dared to ask the question, "What is the typical life "runway" of a resident at a memory care with this ugly disease?" The response was not one I wanted to hear, but statistically it is about *one year* from the time they are admitted. The reason for this incredibly short span of life is due to the nature of the disease and the time it takes us as caregivers to decide to relocate our loved-ones—usually toward the end or final phase of the disease.

Alzheimer's and dementia are always in a downward spiral. Like a whirlpool, plunging faster and deeper, speeding up as the severity of the disease brings our loved ones closer to the end of life.

We wait as long as we can endure to have them at our side at home, no matter how painful that may be. Typically, in what is medically the final stage of this ugly disease we relocate them. This spiraling downward is something that is never fully appreciated by the caregiver until we see it in our rearview mirror. The timeline is not a straight-line. It bends decidedly downward, and very quickly the closer we get to the end.

The residents at any memory care facility are at best a mix bag of symptoms and behaviors. Some will break the statistical averages and live for several years. They have a *longer runway*, particularly, since those with Alzheimer's and dementia are increasingly getting the disease at a younger age—in their 60's and 70's, with a few even in their 50's. Others, however, are overtaken by the disease with their age and perhaps with other medical issues that will align with the statistical average. If we are not realistic about life, and about death, *end of life* will catch us by surprise—it will come sooner than we expect, or, perhaps, sooner than we want. This is the ultimate certainty about *waiting*.

One of the reoccurring questions I am asked by the hospice assessment staff and by the staff of the memory care facility is, *"Do you have end-of-life plans in place for your loved one?"* My typical answer is "No, not yet." After all, it was about all I could do just to get my wife relocated to memory care. *End of life plans*—well, that is for another day, month or year. However we think about it, it is just not *immediate* in our thinking. Even as I was reviewing the draft for this chapter, the hospice chaplain called to see if I needed help in making plans for my wife's end-of-life interment. What do they know about what I am obviously neglecting, ignoring or denying?

A recent candid conversation with the hospice case manager only brought the reality of *waiting* into focus. "The end-of-life," she said, "will come sooner than you expect." She went on to explain my wife's condition and said that her last three falls have only accelerated her decline—they have shortened her "runway"—her life-expectancy. "Be ready!" was the case manager's caution. Within the space of a month, Beverley went from being reasonably ambulatory to being confined to a high-back wheelchair. Within a six-month period, she went from being one who could wear a beautiful smile to one who is a silent victim of this ugly disease. I went from a loving caregiver who blissfully considered that the decline would take several years before the end-of-life came, to one who has been forced to make end-of-life interment plans, *now. Waiting?* Yes, but for how long?

Unhappily, as a loving spouse or child, we need to include such thinking and planning into our *waiting.* If you have hospice, talk about this subject with the social worker assigned to your case or the hospice chaplain. Engage the family, no matter how difficult it may be to talk about *end-of-life plans* for your loved one. Visit a local funeral home and begin a conversation with them. Select a cemetery. Is your loved one a veteran, or a spouse that can qualify for VA burial benefits? The more you do now will make a very difficult period of *waiting* easier. It is much less stressful to plan these things "now" rather than at the time of death.

However, there is more to *waiting* than just waiting for the end of life of our loved one. Without the one who has been at my side for 55 years, I am now learning to wait by *occupying*—creating new spaces for myself to become a loving husband who can superintend at an emotional distance. In Bev's new living environment, I still care for her needs, but much of the time it is through the hands of a professionally trained staff.

Here's what I found. The more time I spent at the memory care facility the less time I had emotionally in becoming the loving spouse I needed to be. With my frequent visits, I found that I was still trying to be a caregiver. I needed to change my attitude. I want to be careful here. I am not encouraging abandonment of our loved one—just determine what the right balance is for you and your loved one in a very difficult situation. It's a process of adapting our behavior to what is becoming real in the life of our loved one, i.e., they are becoming less dependent on us.

As newly unfettered caregivers, we must learn to wait and to *wait well.* Transitioning from a caregiver to a loving spouse or devoted child is difficult and can be painful. But now is the time to discover (or rediscover) the person that is you. Discover who you are socially, unearth your passions—what are the things that excite you; how about those interests and talents you laid aside over the years? It is time for you to awaken them and to move on into your new single life.

It is not wrong—*you are not dishonoring your relationship with your loved one* to start again to enjoy the sweetness and beauty of life, whether that means travel, planting a garden or engaging in some civic or church-related activity, or all of the above. Taking an occasional afternoon nap—with *both eyes closed*—is also on the list of discovering something new. These discoveries are all part of this time we call, *waiting*. All the while we continue to honor the one we love.

These things will help form you *again* into the loving spouse or devoted child your loved one needs at this most critical, but special time in their lives and yours.

****

Afterthoughts

In seven brief chapters we have made our journey into the deepest struggles of the caregiver of *this ugly disease*—the depths of which the average person rarely has any comprehension. Some have suggested that the seven chapters be developed and expanded into a *book*. But, no. While there is sufficient content yet to be discussed and interviews to be recorded, I am writing this *booklet* for the caregiver. In their pain and anguish of doing what is beyond human limits and endurance, they do not have time to read *a book*. They will be challenged just to pick up this small booklet and try to focus on seven brief chapters. What I want for each of them, and for you, is to be encouraged and grab some hope along the way.

For the most part, I have left the "how-to" of caregiving to many excellent books written on the mechanics of caregiving. My heart's desire is to assure and comfort the caregiver that *they are not alone* in their frustrations and inadequacies, in their times of emotional breakdowns, and in feeling they can no longer provide the care their loved one needs.

In our utter desperation there is a beacon of hope. *Help* is available, if only we know where, how and when to ask for it. That is what this little booklet seeks to provide. There is also hope in becoming again *a new you* as you seek to be the loving spouse or devoted child for your loved one.

One more thing, I have added a final word. I want to share with you, as caregiver to caregiver, how my faith, the spiritual bucket, is for me a "must-have" as an essential part of the journey.

A Final Word

Faith

Faith is a very elusive thing, particularly for a caregiver. We have it, yet we don't. Faith has not failed us—God remains faithful, but how many times have we failed our faith? How many times did we forget that God was part of the journey? Hammered by guilt and untold misbehaviors, how many times did we need to say, "Father, I have sinned," —over and over, even for the same thing?

Caregiving, when I take it to my ultimate human limits, reveals the darker side of my nature. I would like to believe that with maturity and the wisdom of age, my nature has improved. But caregiving quickly and with clarity shows me how *unimproved* I really am. It lays bare all the grossness of the human spirit when put to the wall. Maybe your experience was different, but this was mine.

Stripping aside all the niceties most people know about us, here is what I found. At the core of my nature, given the right set of circumstances provided easily to every caregiver, I am as ugly as the disease I hate. I will spare the details already discussed in a previous chapter. We as caregivers understand these behaviors all too well.

Throughout this booklet I refer to my *spiritual bucket*. This resource, along with my physical, mental and emotional buckets, ran dry. It was a terrible feeling! At the top level of my brain I knew what I needed to do, but the top level of my brain was not functioning. It was being daily overwhelmed by gut-wrenching turmoil buried deep within my soul. I knew deep inside I was running on empty.

Here is something else I found. Caregiving and faith are inseparable. I am not really sure how people do the job of caregiving without an element of faith—that in the middle of our confusion and chaos there remains the God who orders and controls events beyond our ability. The One who is supremely more concerned about our loved one than we could ever be!

Having trusted Jesus as my Savior and Lord, and having the Holy Spirit as my Comforter—these are all helps beyond description. Iam not ashamed to say that cannot make it through life without the Lord and the hope He gives for eternal life after this life on earth has passed. This was Beverley's hope as well. It is good to remember that God does not always prevent us from going through trials. However, He promises to be with us as we go through them. Even in this journey of Bev's dementia—*this ugly disease*, I can affirm His faithfulness.

Orchestrating the times and events of my *tragic opera,* He began to shine light into the dark recesses of my spiritual bucket. He reminded me of His *absolute* love and *perfect* forgiveness that has never wavered. I soon realized that He did not change one iota throughout the mess I was in. It was I who changed.

Eyes often wet with tears of anguish and frustration, of remorse and confusion, I now feel like a wreck of an old wooden vessel emerging from a terrible storm at sea, with sails torn and a broken mast—emerging into the sunlight.

Recently, my son dropped into my computer a couple of verses to a very old German Lutheran hymn that for me was faith renewing. I hope you find it to be so:

Be still, my soul: the Lord is on thy side.

Bear patiently the cross of grief or pain.

Leave to thy God to order and provide;

In every change, He faithful will remain.

Be still, my soul: thy best, thy heav'nly Friend

Through thorny ways leads to a joyful end.

Be still, my soul: thy God doth undertake

To guide the future, as He has the past.

Thy hope, thy confidence let nothing shake;

All now mysterious shall be bright at last.

Be still, my soul: the waves and winds still know

His voice Who ruled them while He dwelt below.

Kathrina von Schlegel (1752)
Translated: Jane L. Borthwick (1855)
(Public Domain)

Based upon Lamentations 3:19-24

[19]*I remember my affliction and my wandering,*

the bitterness and the gall.

[20]*I well remember them,*

and my soul is downcast within me.

[21]*Yet this I call to mind*

and therefore I have hope:

[22]*Because of the Lord's great love we are not consumed,*

for his compassions never fail.

[23]*They are new every morning;*

great is your faithfulness.

[24]*I say to myself, "The Lord is my portion;*

therefore I will wait for him.

An Addendum

A Lost Ring – The End of A Journey

The phone rang just before bedtime. The call was from the memory care facility where Beverley lives. I dreaded those calls because I knew what I would hear. "Your wife has fallen—*again*."

This was the fifth fall, but not the last. Like all falls, it was serious—another concussion to the head. Trying to determine the extent of the wound and if the night staff had called the hospice nurse, I noticed that my ring was missing from my finger—the wedding band that I had worn for 55 years was gone. In the days that followed, I searched everywhere—in the bed, under it, around it, and everywhere else I could think of. No ring!

The fall made a significant impact on Bev's behavior. Her responses declined, and she no longer swallowed regular food. The nurse placed her on a soft food/liquid diet. Initially, she adapted to the new diet but soon pushed back. Sometimes eating and drinking, other times taking nothing.

What I discovered is a person's departure is not always a straight line to the end. This was the case with Beverley—it may be for your loved one as well. Her journey to the end was marked by ups and downs—a roller coaster of changing behaviors but always heading in the same direction. Be careful not to be too excited about your loved one's improved behavior. A peak, yes, but a deep valley will follow quickly. The body is shutting down. It's a matter of time.

The "ups and downs" of this extended final journey can be terribly hard on the family. But remember, each day provides precious opportunities for saying goodbye. Whatever kind of day it is, receive it as a special gift to spend time with your loved one in their final days. Eventually, their hearing may be impaired, but a gentle caress to the cheek or forehead is a "word" that always speaks, that is always "heard."

Be sure to give opportunity for closure to your loved one and to others in the immediate family. If they cannot come to the bedside to express their love, say their goodbyes and give your loved one permission to depart this life, then use the available technology of iPhones, Face-Time, Skype, etc.

In her final hours, Bev resisted leaving us until her three sons said their goodbye's. I used Face-Time on my iPad to allow each of our two sons to say their goodbye's and to assure their mother that they would all be okay. To say she was free to go *home*! From North Carolina, the youngest son said his loving goodbye. The second oldest son said his goodbye from Kansas—he even sang a farewell love-song to her. My oldest son and I were at her bedside as we said goodbye and placed a loving kiss on her forehead, while holding her hand. Within a few minutes she quietly slipped into a deep coma. Within a few short hours she left us.

If there are outstanding issues of emotional distance and separation among family members, although not always easy, it is a beautiful time to reconcile these differences. Life at best is short indeed!

Memories of my times with Bev at the memory care center began to flow into my mind. I remembered how She continued to recognize who I was. At every visit I would ask if she knew who I was. Until she could longer speak, she would always say, "Don." I would respond by saying, "I love you." I shared pictures on my iPad of roses with her—her favorite flower. Again, I asked her to name the flower. She did, "roses." I remember, too, even though she could no longer speak or barely move, at every meal time she motioned to the staff that she wanted to set next to the same person at the table. That person could not feed himself and would need to wait until meal time was over until a staff person could feed him. Not sure how she did, but Bev fed him! That's who she was!

Not once did she complain by word or by expression about her situation either in the memory care facility or in the years before. Because of family history, she understood for many years that one day this ugly disease would bring her to heaven and her Lord. All who saw her, both staff and visitors, said she was a woman at peace. In her own way, she conquered this ugly disease by making peace with it.

Beverley's sixth fall came within two weeks of her previous one. A few days after the fall, almost comatose, she sat sleeping in her wheelchair, only occasionally opening her eyes, staring at nothing. Eating nothing. Drinking nothing. For her safety, the nurse recommended that she be bed-bound most of the time. Eventually, her complexion turned ashen and her condition became catatonic. Within a few days, her journey into this ugly disease was coming to an end. Struggling to breath normally, she was placed on continuous care— under a 24/7 hospice nurse watch. About mid-night on February 15th she peacefully ended her journey. *I had lost my ring, but now I lost my wife.*

Bev ended her journey, not as a defeated victim of dementia but as a faithful servant of her Lord, joyfully going home to be embraced by Him and to receive a victor's crown as her reward. She is now free from the bondage and shackles of her nemesis. No longer does she struggle with a mind and body that imprisoned her spirit from expressing fully who she is. Her faith firmly rooted in Jesus, she is now with Him, which is always far better.

Knowing this about Beverley, however, does not mean there is no sadness, sorrow or a period of grieving for those left behind who must still sort through the leftover pieces of this journey.

The time of "letting go" and "waiting" discussed in Chapters 6 and 7 is over. After all is done, there remains the *sound of silence*. Each of us deals with grief uniquely. Sometimes it is lengthy; sometimes short, but a scar remains. Hopefully, each of us finds the coping process that helps us work through it. Grief is something to be managed, or it will manage us; it is a healthy part of living.

I am reminded that Jesus grieved at the loss of his friend, Lazarus, but still provided hope by reminding those around him that He is *the Resurrection and the Life* and that He is caring—He grieves in our loss:

Jesus said to her, "I am the resurrection and the life. Whoever believes in me, though he die, yet shall he live". . . And he said, "Where have you laid him?" They said to him, "Lord, come and see." Jesus wept. (John 11:25, 33-35)

46

Resources

The Alzheimer Association   http://www.alzfdn.org
A rich website filled with information and helps about Alzheimer's and dementia – worth the visit and discovery. Local chapters are listed.

Toll Free Helpline: 866-232-8484 (9am – 9pm EST)

2014 Alzheimer's Disease Facts and Figures
http://www.alz.org/downloads/facts_figures_2014.pdf

Alzheimer's Foundation of America   http://www.alzfdn.org)
There are many books available on the Alzheimer Foundation of America website:

The 36-Hour Day

A Family Guide to Caring for People with Alzheimer Disease, Other Dementias, and Memory Loss in Later Life (September, 2012).
By Nancy L. Mace, M.A.,and Peter V. Rabins, M.D., M.P.H.

Don't Eat The Elephants (May, 2006) by Patricia H. Miller

Alzheirmer's Disease Education and Referral Center
https://www.nia.nih.gov/alzheimers/

Alzheimer's Fact Sheets
https://www.nia.nih.gov/alzheimers/publication?sort_by=totalcount

A Place for Mom   http://www.aplaceformom.com
A good resource for finding appropriate places to locate your loved one, and to keep current on relevant issues from their blog.

Still Alice, available as a *novel or movie on DVD.* December, 2014.
by Lisa Genova
Although framed within a novel, its depiction of dementia is accurate and moving. It is well worth the price. Available at Amazon.com.

Your Comments are always welcomed.
dhzoller@outlook.com

Nine Things I Found Important

They May Help You, Too

1. Recognize you are not alone – Millions of caregivers share your experience.

2. Get professional help – You can't do caregiving on your own.

3. Learn to forgive yourself – Often!

4. Take care of yourself – Physically, mentally, emotionally and spiritually.

5. Get involved in a caregivers' support group.

6. Be informed – Read all you can about Alzheimer's and dementia.

7. Keep a daily journal – It will help you and your family.

8. Be available to help others – Many are traveling the same road.

9. Shake off the dust – become again the loving devoted spouse or child your loved one needs.

www.ingramcontent.com/pod-product-compliance
Lightning Source LLC
Chambersburg PA
CBHW050522290526
45786CB00007B/2656